Tujchiev Rashidbek Valizhon ugli

PECULIARITIES OF PREPARATION FOR ORTHOPEDIC TREATMENT

Tujchiev Rashidbek Valizhon ugli

PECULIARITIES OF PREPARATION FOR ORTHOPEDIC TREATMENT

WITH SECONDARY DENTAL DEFORMITIES

ScienciaScripts

Cover image: www.ingimage.com

This book is a translation from the original published under ISBN 978-620-8-41755-0.

Publisher:
Sciencia Scripts
is a trademark of
Dodo Books Indian Ocean Ltd. and OmniScriptum S.R.L publishing group

120 High Road, East Finchley, London, N2 9ED, United Kingdom
Str. Armeneasca 28/1, office 1, Chisinau MD-2012, Republic of Moldova, Europe
Managing Directors: Ieva Konstantinova, Victoria Ursu
info@omniscriptum.com

Printed at: see last page
ISBN: 978-620-8-61447-8

Tujchiev Rashidbek Valizhon ugli

PECULIARITIES OF PREPARATION FOR ORTHOPAEDIC TREATMENT OF SECONDARY DENTAL DEFORMITIES

Monograph

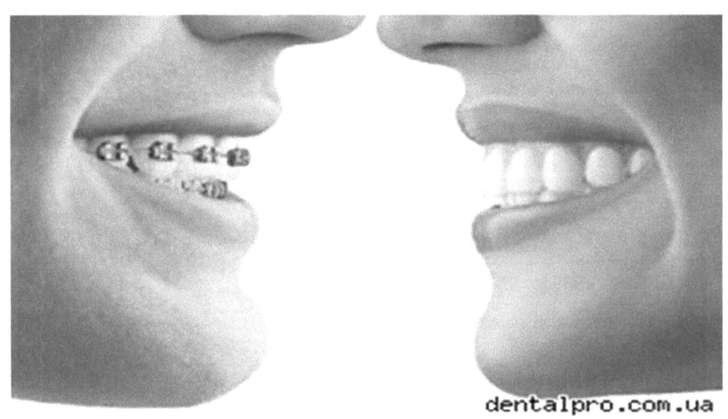

PECULIARITIES OF PREPARATION FOR ORTHOPAEDIC TREATMENT WITH SECONDARY DENTAL DEFORMITIES.

Contents.

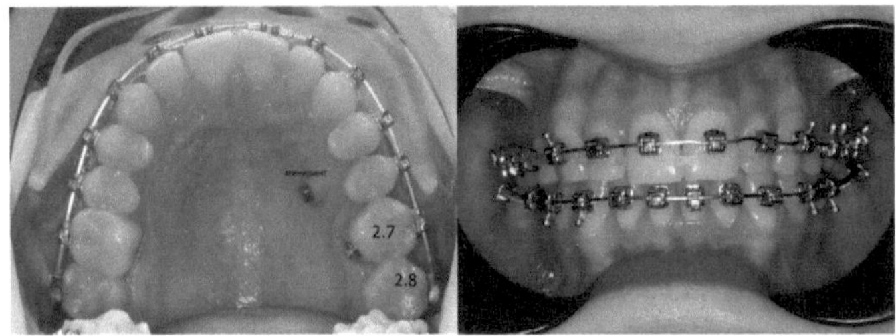
2.7
2.8

Introduction

Preparation for orthopaedic treatment of patients with secondary dental deformities is one of the most difficult and responsible tasks of modern dentistry. Secondary deformities are changes in the structure and function of the dento-mandibular system resulting from pathological processes or lack of timely treatment. These changes include displacement of teeth, violation of occlusion and aesthetics, as well as bone atrophy. Their treatment requires a comprehensive approach aimed at restoring chewing efficiency, aesthetics and preventing further complications.

Relevance of the topic

Modern dentistry is faced with an increasing number of patients suffering from the consequences of secondary dental deformities. This is due to the growing number of periodontal diseases, increasing life expectancy and, as a consequence, the need for long-term preservation of the functionality of the dento-mandibular system. Also of considerable importance are the consequences of trauma and dental treatment errors, which cause complex clinical cases.

Restoration of anatomical integrity of the dentition and masticatory function is a key prerequisite for maintaining the general health of patients, including the prevention of gastrointestinal diseases, temporomandibular joint disorders, and even systemic diseases. Thus, the issues of preparation for orthopaedic treatment of patients with secondary dental deformities are becoming an important area of scientific research and practical dentistry.

Aim and objectives of the study

Purpose of the study: Development and justification of a comprehensive approach to the diagnosis, preparation and treatment of patients with secondary dental deformities.

Objectives of the study:

1. to study the main causes and mechanisms of development of secondary dental deformities.

2. To analyse modern diagnostic methods and their application in clinical practice.

3. Develop a classification of secondary deformities that takes into account etiological and morphological aspects.

4. to study the peculiarities of preparation of the dento-mandibular system for orthopaedic treatment.

5. To develop recommendations on the choice of treatment methods depending on the severity of deformities.

6. To evaluate the effectiveness of interdisciplinary approach in complex rehabilitation of patients.

Research methodology

The following methods were used to achieve the objectives:

- Analysis of scientific literature and current data on the problem of secondary deformities of the dentition.

- Clinical studies involving the examination of patients with different types of deformities.

- Application of instrumental diagnostic methods (orthopantomography, cone-beam computed tomography, occlusographic analysis).

- Evaluation of treatment outcomes using statistical methods of analysis.

Scientific novelty and practical significance

A new approach to the classification of secondary deformities has been developed within the framework of the study, allowing to take into account their complex pathogenetic mechanisms and clinical manifestations. Improved methods of preparing the dento-mandibular system for orthopaedic treatment based on the use of modern technologies, including 3D modelling and digital planning, have been proposed. The obtained data can be used to develop diagnostic and treatment standards, which will increase the efficiency and predictability of orthopaedic rehabilitation.

Structure of the work

This monograph consists of an introduction, five chapters, a conclusion, and a list of references. The first chapter deals with the causes and classification of secondary deformities of the dentition. The second chapter deals with modern diagnostic methods. The third chapter is devoted to the main stages of preparation for orthopaedic treatment. The fourth and fifth chapters discuss the peculiarities of treatment and rehabilitation of patients.

This monograph is aimed at dental specialists, orthopaedists and medical students interested in modern approaches to the diagnosis and treatment of secondary dental deformities.

Chapter 1: Secondary dental deformities: causes and classification

1.1 Causes of secondary deformations

Secondary dental deformities are changes in the structure and function of the dentoalveolar system that arise and develop under the influence of various factors. These changes can be due to both internal (endogenous) and external (exogenous) causes affecting the teeth, periodontium and bone tissue.

1.1.1 Endogenous causes

1. **Age-related changes:**
    - **Decreased bone density.** In older adults, there is a natural weakening of bone structure, especially in the jaw area, which makes teeth more vulnerable to movement and loss. Bone tissue loses its density, which can contribute to a redistribution of stress on the teeth, as well as changes in their position.
    - **Physiological tooth erosion.** With age, the natural erosion of enamel occurs, which disturbs the occlusal contact (the correct relationship between the upper and lower teeth). This can lead to misalignment of the teeth, development of tooth tilt, and gaps between the teeth.
    - **Changes in blood vessels and nerve endings.** As we age, the vascular system and nerves that supply the teeth and gums become less elastic, which affects tissue nutrition and repair. This can cause changes in the teeth and periodontium, contributing to tooth misalignment and deformities.
2. **Genetic factors:**

- **Hereditary predisposition.** Genetic predisposition plays an important role in the development of periodontal diseases such as paradontitis and bite abnormalities. People whose relatives have suffered from such diseases are more likely to have the same problems.
- **Peculiarities of the structure of the maxillofacial apparatus.** Genetic factors can lead to abnormal jaw size, which in turn can affect the positioning of the teeth. For example, a narrow jaw or teeth that are too large can cause them to become crooked, tilted, or overly compressed.
- **Soft tissue underdevelopment or hypertrophy.** Abnormalities in the development of soft tissues, such as gingiva or ligaments, can also be genetically determined and affect the stability of teeth, leading to tooth movement and deformity.

3. **Metabolic disorders:**
   - **Vitamin and mineral deficiencies.** Deficiencies of vital elements such as calcium, vitamin D and phosphorus affect bone and tooth strength. Decreased levels of these substances can weaken the bones of the jaw, which in turn increases the risk of dental deformities and tooth loss. For example, calcium deficiency makes teeth more susceptible to breaking and shifting.
   - **Endocrine diseases.** Various diseases of the endocrine system such as diabetes, hypo- and hyperthyroidism can cause inflammation in periodontal tissue and bone. Changes in the levels of hormones such as insulin, thyroxine or calcitonin can affect bone mineralisation and dental health. For example, diabetes increases susceptibility to infection

and inflammation, which can contribute to periodontal disease and resulting changes in tooth position.

- **Hormonal fluctuations.** Hormonal changes, such as those that occur during pregnancy, menopause, or adolescence, can significantly affect gum and bone health, making them more prone to inflammation and tooth loss. In menopausal women, decreased estrogen levels can affect bone strength, increasing the risk of osteoporosis and worsening periodontal health.

4. **Psycho-emotional factors:**
   - **Stress and nervous disorders.** Psycho-emotional stress can cause tension in the muscles of the jaw, which interferes with the normal function of the dentoalveolar system. Chronic stress can also contribute to bruxism (teeth grinding), which leads to increased tooth wear and misalignment.
   - **Chronic fatigue syndrome.** Individuals suffering from chronic fatigue may experience changes in the immune system, which increases the propensity for oral inflammation and periodontal deterioration.

All of this comes together to create a comprehensive picture of the factors that influence the stability and health of the dentition at different ages.

1.1.2 Exogenous causes affecting the structure and functionality of the dento-mandibular system

Exogenous causes affecting the dentoalveolar system are external factors that can lead to the development of secondary dental deformities. These causes can be related to trauma, disease, improper treatment, and socioeconomic aspects. Let us consider the main exogenous factors affecting the dento-mandibular system.

1. **Tooth loss and associated occlusal changes:**
   - **Loss of one or more teeth.** When teeth are lost, especially in the anterior or masseter, neighbouring and antagonistic teeth begin to move, which disturbs the overall balance of the dentition. Neighbouring teeth begin to migrate towards the defect, causing changes in interdental contacts and contributing to the deformity of the dentition.

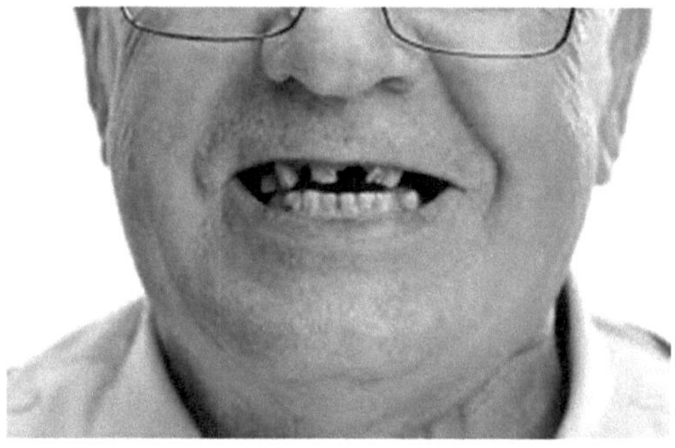

   - **Changes in occlusion.** Occlusal defects (e.g. malocclusion) are associated with tooth loss and migration of neighbouring teeth, which disrupts the natural relationship of the tooth rows. Tooth misalignment can lead to temporomandibular joint (TMJ) dysfunction and can cause problems with chewing and speech.

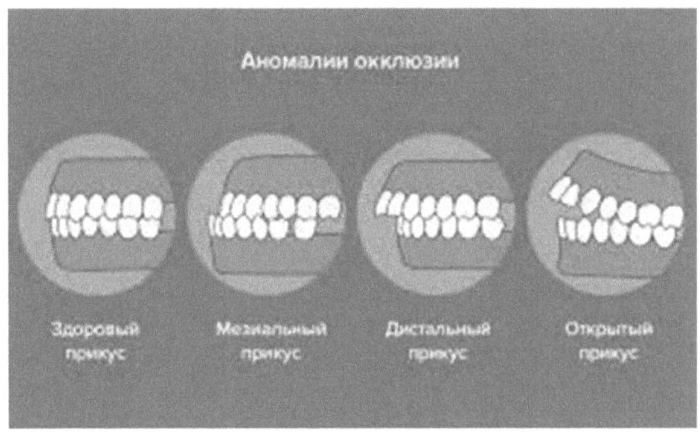

- **Atrophy of the alveolar process.** The lack of masticatory load in the defect areas contributes to bone atrophy in the area of the dentition. This can impair the conditions for fitting dentures or implants and lead to further changes in the position of the teeth.

2. **Periodontal Diseases:**
   - **Inflammatory diseases.** Gingivitis and periodontitis are inflammatory processes that are accompanied by destruction of periodontal tissues (gums, ligaments, bone tissue), which leads to increased tooth mobility and migration. These diseases disturb the stability of teeth and can lead to their loss.
   - **Progressive bone resorption.** As a result of inflammation in the periodontal tissues, there is a gradual destruction of the bone tissue of the jaw, which aggravates the migration of teeth and impairs the fixation of teeth in the alveoli. This can lead to tooth loss and tooth displacement in the dentition.
   - **Decreased tooth support.** Due to bone resorption and damage to periodontal ligaments, teeth become more

mobile, which contributes to their displacement. This also increases the likelihood of secondary occlusal defects and disorders of the entire dentoalveolar system.

- 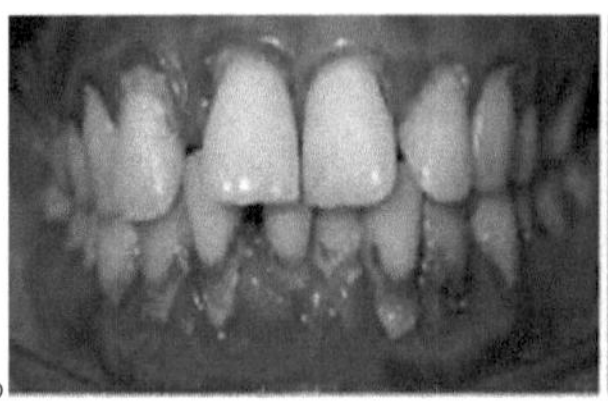 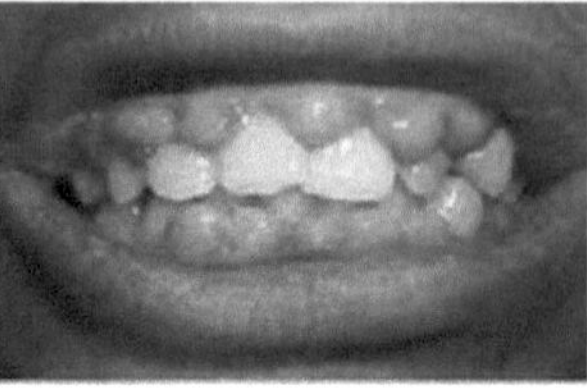

3. **Errors and complications of dental treatment:**
    - **Poor-quality dentures and implants.** An improperly fitted denture or implant that compromises contact points or occlusion can lead to tooth misalignment and impaired function. Poor workmanship, such as in the fabrication of dentures, can disrupt the biomechanics of the dentoalveolar system and cause secondary deformities.
    - **Incorrect orthodontic treatment.** Errors in orthodontic treatment (e.g. incorrect planning or inappropriate selection of orthodontic appliances) can lead to improper distribution of the load on the teeth, which in turn contributes to changes in their position and deformities in the dentition. It can also cause joint problems such as TMJ dysfunction.
4. **Improper distribution of chewing load:**
    - **Defects in the dentition.** If there are defects in the dentition, such as missing teeth, incorrect dentures or orthodontic anomalies, the load on the teeth is not evenly distributed. This can contribute to wear and tear and can also lead to the development of abnormal tooth erosion, which contributes to tooth misalignment and deformation.
    - **Overloading.** When individual teeth are subjected to excessive pressure (e.g., with an improper bite or after

dentures), this accelerates their wear and can also cause them to tilt or shift, creating conditions for secondary dental deformities.

5. **Socio-economic factors:**
   - **Lack of access to quality dental care.** In some regions or for certain segments of the population, limited access to high quality dental care can lead to delays in the diagnosis and treatment of diseases of the dento-mandibular system. This can lead to dental deterioration, tooth loss and the development of secondary deformities.
   - **Neglect of preventive measures.** Lack of attention to the prevention of dental diseases, lack of regular check-ups with a dentist, inadequate oral hygiene can lead to the development of periodontal and dental diseases, which creates the conditions for deformities. Also, lack of preventive measures can contribute to the accumulation of dental plaque, which is the main risk factor for the development of dental caries and periodontal diseases.
6. **Traumatic injuries:**
   - **Mechanical trauma to the jaw or teeth.** Injuries such as blows or fractures to the jaw or teeth can lead to misalignment and damage to dental structures. Tooth fractures or compromised bone integrity often result in tooth loss, which disrupts the overall balance of the dentoalveolar system and can cause migration of neighbouring teeth.
   - **Consequences of trauma.** After trauma, teeth may be displaced or even lost, contributing to occlusal defects and secondary deformities. For example, if the jaw or teeth are fractured, improper treatment or lack of timely

rehabilitation can exacerbate the situation and lead to long-term changes in the dentoalveolar system.

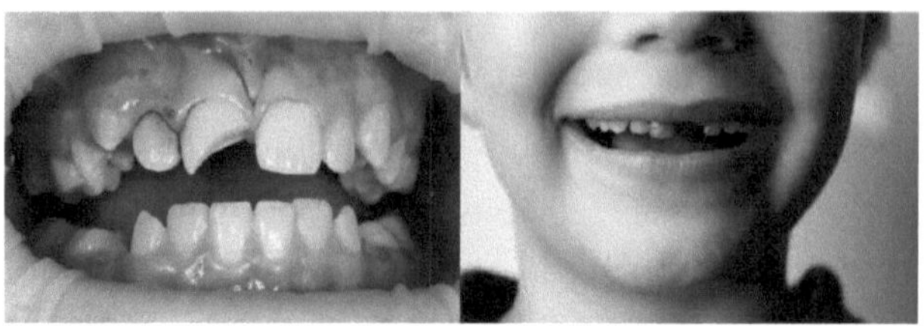

7. **Errors and complications following dental interventions:**
   - **Poor quality work during orthodontic treatment.** Errors in the process of installing braces or other orthodontic appliances that do not take into account the peculiarities of the patient's anatomy can lead to improper tooth movement. This, in turn, will cause deformation of the tooth row and change its position.
   - **Iatrogenic factors.** These factors include errors associated with improperly fabricated fillings, crowns or bridges that can interfere with contact points and lead to changes in occlusion. An improperly fitted denture can affect the teeth and jaws in a way that causes them to shift or deform.

Thus, exogenous factors can significantly affect the stability and functionality of the dento-mandibular system, leading to secondary deformities of the dentition, occlusion disorders and deterioration of teeth and periodontal tissues.

1.2 Classification of secondary deformations.

Classification of secondary dental deformities allows systematising data on pathological changes, highlighting their features and causes.

This is important for making a diagnosis and selecting treatment tactics.

For ease of diagnosis and choice of treatment tactics, secondary dental deformities are classified according to the following criteria:**1.2.1.**

1. **By localisation:**
   - Frontal deformities (incisors and canines).
   - Deformities of the masseter (premolars and molars).
2. **In terms of severity:**
   - Minor (initial occlusal changes that do not require significant intervention).
   - Moderate (displacement of teeth, changes in chewing efficiency).
   - Severe (significant occlusion disorder requiring complex treatment).
3. **Etiology:**
   - Traumatic (consequences of mechanical injuries).
   - Inflammatory (related to periodontal disease.
4. Iatrogenic:
   - Due to complications of treatment or poorly performed medical procedures.a).
   - Iatrogenic (the result of poor-quality treatment or doctor's errors).
5. **By nature of changes:**Horizontal (movement of
   - Horizontal (displacement of teeth in anteroposterior direction).
   - Vertical (intrusion or extrusion).
   - Rotational (tooth rotations).
   - Vertical (extrusion or intrusion of teeth).
   - Rotational (turning the teeth around their axis).

6. **Functional consequences:** Disorder of occlusion.
7. Aesthetic defects.
   - Occlusal disorders.
   - Aesthetic defects.
   - Combined.
8. **In terms of the duration of the deformation:**
   - Acute (recent onset).
   - Chronic (long-term).

1.3 Biomechanical aspects of secondary deformations

Biomechanical aspects of secondary dental deformities encompass the interaction of various structures of the dentoalveolar system and the influence of various factors on the stability of teeth and their position. These aspects are of key importance in understanding the mechanisms of development of secondary deformities, as well as in selecting effective methods of their treatment and prevention.

1. **An imbalance between the teeth and the chewing muscles:**
   - Normally, the dentoalveolar system works in harmony between the teeth, bone tissue, gums and masticatory muscles. When this equilibrium is disturbed, e.g. due to changes in tooth position, incorrect distribution of the chewing load or occlusal defects, certain muscles become overstretched. This can cause the teeth to shift towards the defect or create conditions for them to tilt and change position. Such imbalances can also lead to additional stresses on the TMJ (temporomandibular joint), which contributes to pain and other functional disorders.
2. **The influence of occlusal contacts:**

- Occlusion is the relationship of the tooth rows when the teeth are compressed. Improper occlusal contacts create areas of overload on individual teeth, which can cause their displacement or abnormal loading on bone structures. For example, when interdental contacts are inappropriate (e.g., improper bite or missing teeth), teeth may be subjected to additional pressure, which accelerates their migration or causes misalignment of the tooth rows. Improper occlusion can also contribute to excessive tooth wear or bruxism (teeth grinding), which further aggravates the situation.

3. **The role of bone tissue:**
   - **Alveolar atrophy.** Bone atrophy in the area of a defect (e.g. tooth loss) is an important biomechanical process that directly affects the stability of the remaining teeth. Without load on certain areas of the jaw, e.g. at the site of a missing tooth, the alveolar process begins to atrophy, reducing the supporting function for the neighbouring teeth. This creates conditions for their displacement and further changes in the tooth row. Thus, bone atrophy exacerbates the problem of tooth loss, contributing to the migration of neighbouring teeth and worsening the overall position of the dentoalveolar system.
4. **An interdisciplinary approach:**
   - In order to effectively treat secondary dental deformities, it is important to take into account data from different medical disciplines. A combined approach that includes orthodontics, orthopaedics and oral surgery can properly assess and treat the causes of deformities. For example, an orthodontist can correct misaligned teeth with braces or other appliances, while an orthopedist can restore lost teeth

with dentures or implants. Surgery may be required to rebuild bone and correct jaw deformities to help prevent further migration of teeth and stabilise their position. This comprehensive approach ensures the best possible outcome and minimises the risk of deformity recurrence.

1.4 Social and psychological aspects

Secondary dental deformities not only affect the physical condition of the patient, but can also have significant social and psychological consequences. Changes in the dentoalveolar system can affect the patient's quality of life, self-confidence and social adaptation.

1. **Aesthetic discomfort:**
   - Tooth misalignment and occlusal defects such as crossing, misalignment or gaps between teeth can significantly affect the aesthetics of the smile. Aesthetic problems cause psychological discomfort for the patient, as appearance plays an important role in social life. People with deformed teeth often feel self-conscious, avoid socialising and limit their participation in social events, which can affect their self-esteem and self-confidence.
2. **Social adaptation:**
   - Changes in appearance, including changes in the dentoalveolar system, can make it difficult for patients to adapt socially, especially if the defects affect speech or facial expression. People with dentoalveolar disorders may experience difficulties in interpersonal communication and may also face problems in their professional and personal lives. This can lead to social isolation, depression and even reduced ability to work.

3. **The importance of patient information:**
    - Informing patients about the causes of secondary deformities and the possible consequences of these changes is important to increase their motivation for treatment. Patients who understand the importance of early diagnosis and prevention of dentoalveolar disorders are more likely to participate in treatment and follow the dentist's recommendations. Explaining all stages of treatment, including possible risks and benefits, helps to reduce anxiety and improve patient-doctor interaction.

1.5 Clinical examples and illustrations

Clinical examples and photographs of patients with secondary dental deformities can serve as an excellent tool for visualising the main classifications of deformities and their developmental features. Demonstration of real cases helps:

- Show the variety of secondary deformities: from minor changes in tooth position to more complex cases with disruption of occlusal function and bone structure.
- Evaluate the results of treatment: before and after photos allow you to see how effectively secondary deformities can be corrected with orthodontic or orthopaedic interventions.
- Demonstrate the importance of early intervention: early diagnosis and treatment of secondary deformities significantly increases the chances of successful restoration of the dentition and normalisation of dento-mandibular function.

Clinical cases, supplemented by detailed descriptions of the treatment methods used in each case, illustrate the importance of a comprehensive approach and the correct choice of treatment tactics to achieve the best results.

In-depth discussion of causes and categorisation

Socio-economic factors: Insufficient accessibility of dental care and low level of dental culture of the population play an important role. Neglect of regular preventive care and late seeking of help contribute to the development of complex deformities.1.3 Biomechanical aspects of secondary deformities.

Biomechanical aspects: Displacement of teeth leads to a change in the distribution of loads, which exacerbates existing deformities and creates new problems. Analyses of occlusion and mastication biomechanics play a key role in understanding the processes leading to deformities.

Individual characteristics: Genetic predisposition, age, bone health and regenerative capacity are also important factors in the development of secondary deformities.

Chapter 2: Diagnosis of secondary deformations

Secondary deformities of the dentoalveolar system are the result of various pathological conditions and require careful diagnosis in order to choose the optimal treatment tactics. The diagnostic process involves the use of modern imaging techniques, functional tests and occlusal analysis, which allows specialists to accurately diagnose and predict the progression of the disease. This chapter discusses key techniques for diagnosing secondary deformities and provides case examples.

2.1 Modern diagnostic methods

A number of modern methods are used to diagnose secondary deformities of the dentoalveolar system, which provide accurate information about the condition of the teeth, jaws, soft tissues and other important structures. Key diagnostic methods are described below.

2.1.1 Radiography

Radiography remains one of the most accessible and widely used diagnostic methods in dentistry. Modern radiographic technology allows imaging with minimal radiation dose and high accuracy. The main types of radiography used for the diagnosis of secondary deformities:

1. **Panoramic radiography (orthopantomogram):**
    - This method provides an overview of the entire dento-mandibular system, including the teeth, jaws and temporomandibular joint. Panoramic radiographs are the main tool for initial diagnosis, as they can detect changes in bone structure, inflammatory processes and other pathologies. Panoramic radiography helps in the diagnosis

of various deformities and pathologies such as dental anomalies, periodontal diseases, bone defects and joint diseases.

2. **Cephalometrics:**
   - It is a radiographic method used to evaluate the anatomical characteristics of the skull and its parts, which is particularly important when analysing deformities of the facial and jaw bones. Cephalometric examination allows the position of the teeth and jaws in relation to each other to be assessed, which is important for the diagnosis of occlusal disorders, bite abnormalities, and the detection of abnormalities in normal anatomy.
3. **Radiography in projections:**
   - This method is used when it is necessary to examine specific areas of the jaw, e.g. when deformities or pathological changes are suspected. Images can be taken in different projections to better identify bone destruction, inflammation or signs of traumatic injuries (e.g. osteomyelitis, fractures).

2.1.2 Computed tomography (CT) scanning

Computed tomography (CT) is a high-tech diagnostic method based on layer-by-layer examination, which significantly improves the accuracy of diagnosis of complex deformities and pathologies. CT provides detailed images, which is critical when examining severe secondary deformities.

The use of CT scanning allows:

- Assess bone thickness, bone density and the presence of pathological changes such as bone atrophy, cysts or tumours.
- Examine the condition of the temporomandibular joint, detecting inflammation or degenerative changes.
- Evaluate the spatial relationships between the teeth, jaws, and surrounding soft tissues.
- Plan surgical interventions, especially in complex cases of jaw deformities.

Cone beam computed tomography (CBCT): CBCT is different in that it uses a lower dose of radiation while maintaining high image quality. This is especially important for long-term monitoring of patients with chronic deformities, allowing doctors to track changes over time and adjust treatment. The method is used not only for diagnosis, but also for planning complex dental interventions.

2.1.3 3D modelling

3D modelling is a relatively new technology in diagnosis and treatment planning that allows the creation of accurate three-dimensional images of anatomical structures. The models are created from CT or MRI data and are used for more in-depth analysis of deformities and treatment plans.

Applications of 3D modelling include:

- **Creation of accurate virtual models of jaws and teeth.** These models help specialists to study the mutual arrangement of teeth and jaws in more detail, to identify misalignment of teeth and anomalies in the structure.
- **Surgical modelling.** 3D models make it possible to plan the surgery in advance, assessing its results, which is especially

important in jaw reconstruction or correction of complex deformities.

- **Predicting changes resulting from orthodontic treatment.** Virtual models can predict how teeth will move under the influence of orthodontic appliances, allowing doctors to choose the most appropriate treatment plan and avoid possible complications.

This method is particularly effective when planning complex interventions, such as jaw reconstruction after trauma or disease, and for assessing long-term changes after orthodontic treatment. 3D modelling allows the clinician to visualise the results and evaluate possible intervention options, which significantly improves the treatment outcome.

2.1.4 Functional tests and occlusion analysis

An important part of the diagnosis of secondary deformities is the functional analysis of the dentoalveolar system. It includes:

1. **Assessment of occlusal contacts.** Improper load distribution between the teeth can lead to misalignment. For this, the dentist may use occlusal tests such as impressions with special materials or force probe diagnostics.
2. **Tooth mobility tests.** Tooth mobility often indicates the presence of inflammation in the periodontal tissues as well as progressive bone destruction. To assess tooth mobility, the palpatory method or a special appliance to measure the strength of the mobility can be used.
3. **Masticatory function analysis.** This test helps to detect abnormalities in the temporomandibular joint and masticatory

muscles that may contribute to tooth deformity. Disorders may manifest as pain, restricted movement, or deformed joint surfaces.

2.1.5 Clinical examples

Clinical examples of diagnostic cases help to illustrate the use of different diagnostic methods. Let us consider a few examples:

- **Example 1:** Patient with loss of several teeth and changes in occlusion. The use of panoramic radiography and CT scanning made it possible to assess the state of bone tissue, identify signs of alveolar atrophy and plan prosthetic treatment.

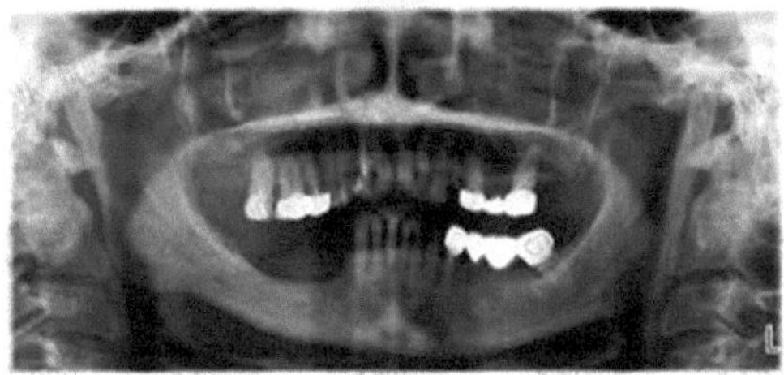

- **Example 2:** Patient with severe jaw deformities after trauma. Cephalometry and 3D modelling allowed to assess the degree of deformity and plan restorative surgery.

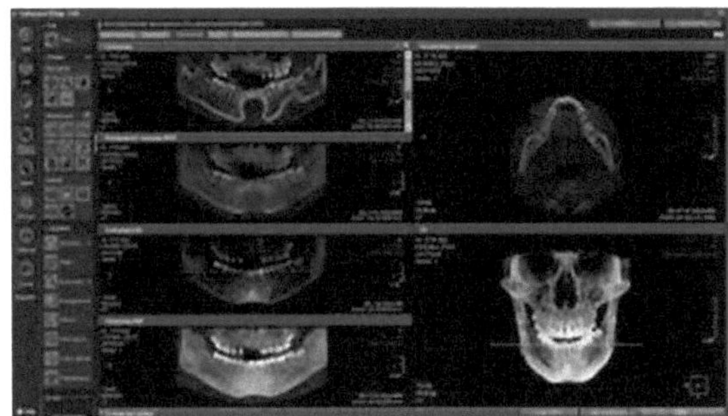

- **Example 3: A** patient with chronic periodontitis and tooth mobility. Functional tests and projection radiographs helped to identify the presence of inflammation and suggested prosthetic treatment with using implants.

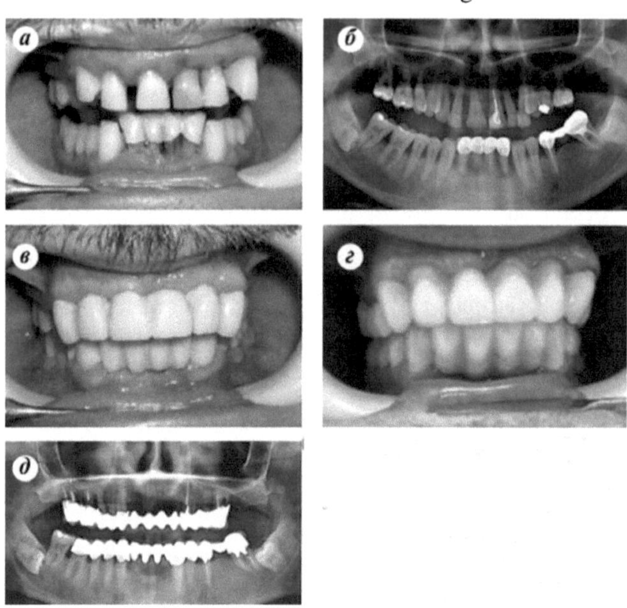

These examples highlight the importance of an integrated approach to diagnosis, where different imaging techniques and functional tests complement each other, allowing accurate diagnoses to be made and effective treatment to be planned.

2.2 Occlusal analyses and functional tests

The occlusal assessment, which is a key element in the diagnosis of secondary deformities, aims to analyse the interaction between the upper and lower jaw teeth. Occlusal abnormalities can be both a cause and a consequence of secondary deformities. It is important to consider that occlusal dysfunction may not only be a factor leading to changes in the dentoalveolar system, but also one of the most important elements in the choice of treatment tactics. This part of the chapter discusses methods for analysing occlusion and functional examinations, which allow for a more accurate diagnosis of problems and the determination of optimal intervention pathways.

2.2.1 Assessment of occlusion

Occlusal evaluation is the process of examining how the upper and lower teeth interact with each other. Several methods are used to do this, which help to identify not only obvious but also hidden abnormalities.

1. **Visual Diagnosis**:
    - This method involves examining the patient in order to detect visible irregularities in the bite. The doctor evaluates the position of the teeth, facial symmetry, jaw relationship and their position relative to each other. Particular attention is paid to crooked teeth, malocclusion, signs of tooth wear and possible temporomandibular joint (TMJ) dysfunction. Visual diagnostics can help identify problems such as malocclusion, open or deep bite, and dental anomalies such as crooked or crowded teeth.
2. **Bite modelling**:
    - This method involves creating accurate impressions of the patient's teeth, which are then analysed to detect abnormalities in their interaction. Bite modelling can detect problems that may not be so obvious at the first examination, but are nevertheless important for diagnosis and treatment planning. The impressions provide an opportunity to examine how the teeth make contact during the different phases of masticatory function and to identify areas of overload or incorrect contact.

3. **Occlusion tests**:
   - These are tests aimed at determining the exact points of tooth contact for various jaw functions such as chewing food, closing the mouth, and making sounds. The doctor may use special paper indicators that mark the contact points of the teeth, as well as functional tests such as bite in motion or static bite analysis. These tests help to detect any irregularities, such as improper load distribution, which can lead to deformation of the dentition.
4. **Digital photogrammetry and computer analyses**:
   - With digital technology, deviations from a normal bite can be measured more accurately. This includes vertical, horizontal and transversal deviations. Modern computer systems can quickly and accurately analyse data obtained from photographs or videos, which helps not only to diagnose abnormalities but also to monitor the dynamics of changes over time. These systems can also build detailed 3D models of the dentition, which facilitates more accurate treatment planning.

2.2.2 Functional studies

Functional examinations play an important role in detecting TMJ pathology and assessing its mobility, as well as in investigating functional disorders that may be associated with occlusal disorders. They allow the detection of hidden problems such as jaw coordination disorders or muscle overstrain, which may lead to secondary deformities.

1. **Electromyography (EMG)**:
   - EMG is an examination method that is used to study the activity of the masticatory muscles. EMG can be used to

assess how much the muscles are tense during the functioning of the dentoalveolar system, as well as to detect the presence of dysfunction that may be associated with TMJ pathology. For example, hypertonicity or underactivity of certain muscles may indicate joint overload or lack of coordination of movements, which may be the cause of secondary deformities.

2. **Rank mobility of the jaw**:
   - This examination method aims to assess the mobility of the jaw in different directions. It helps to detect restrictions or painful jaw movements, which may be due to TMJ damage or arthritis. The mobility study allows you to accurately assess how freely and painlessly the jaw moves in different directions, as well as in which areas of movement pain or restriction occurs.
3. **Articulation overlays and pain tests**:
   - The articulation plates are special devices that allow us to assess the functioning of the TMJ and identify pain syndromes. These plates are placed between the upper and lower teeth to simulate the stresses that the jaws undergo during chewing. In doing so, the doctor can assess the extent to which the joints are stressed and whether there is a pain response. The use of onlays helps to detect functional disorders such as teeth grinding (bruxism) or other disorders that can lead to secondary tooth deformities.
4. **Kinematic studies**:
   - Kinematic studies are one of the most advanced methods for assessing jaw movements. These examinations analyse how the jaw moves during different functions, such as opening and closing the mouth, as well as chewing and pronouncing

sounds. These studies help to identify abnormalities in the coordination of jaw movements as well as TMJ dysfunction. For example, if jaw movements are not synchronised, this can lead to misalignment of teeth, pain and other problems.

Occlusal assessment and functional examinations are the main tools for the diagnosis of secondary deformities of the dentoalveolar system. In combination with imaging and radiographic techniques, these examinations allow clinicians to pinpoint the exact causes of abnormalities and to develop the most effective treatment strategy. It is important that the diagnosis is comprehensive, taking into account all aspects such as the anatomy, physiology and functional characteristics of the dentoalveolar system.

2.3 Clinical examples

Example 1: Traumatic deformity of the mandible

A 36-year-old female patient complained of restricted mobility of the mandible after a car accident. X-ray and CT scans revealed that she had suffered a fracture in the region of the mandibular branch, accompanied by secondary deformation of the bone structure. There was evidence of osteosynthesis, but the mandible was displaced, causing facial asymmetry and bite problems.

After functional tests and occlusion analysis, it was determined that the misalignment of the jaw disrupted the contact between the teeth and also put strain on the temporomandibular joint. Using 3D modelling, surgical correction was planned, after which the patient was offered orthodontic interventions to restore normal occlusion.

Example 2: Secondary deformities in TMJ dysfunction

A 45-year-old patient with chronic pain syndrome in the TMJ area and complaints of difficulty in chewing. According to the results of CT and MRI, a degenerative process in the joint was diagnosed, which was accompanied by inflammation and restricted mobility. Occlusal analysis showed significant bite abnormalities, indicating a link between joint dysfunction and tooth contact disorder.

After functional tests, a decision was made to perform a comprehensive treatment including therapy to relieve TMJ inflammation, occlusion correction using a mouth guard and physiotherapy procedures. The results of treatment demonstrated a significant improvement in functional status.

Thus, the diagnosis of secondary deformities requires the use of modern technologies and techniques, including radiography, CT, 3D modelling, occlusal analysis and functional studies. This allows for accurate diagnosis, development of individualised treatment plans and prediction of possible health consequences for the patient.

Chapter 3: Basic Approaches to Preparing Teeth for Orthopaedic Treatment

The preparation of the dentition for orthopaedic treatment is an important stage that involves a comprehensive approach aimed at restoring both the functionality and aesthetics of the dentoalveolar system. The preparation of the dentition for orthopaedic treatment requires careful attention, detailed diagnosis and close co-operation between specialists from different fields such as dentistry, orthodontics, periodontics and maxillofacial surgery. This chapter details the basic principles of orthopaedic treatment planning, the importance of a multidisciplinary approach, and the role of surgical techniques in the preparation of the dentition.

3.1 Planning principles

Orthopaedic treatment planning is the basis for successful restoration of the maxillary system. It involves a thorough diagnosis, the development of an intervention strategy and the definition of a sequence of treatment measures that will optimally match the patient's individual characteristics, needs and expectations. The more detailed and individualised the treatment plan, the higher the chances of a successful outcome.

3.1.1 Assessment of the clinical situation

The first step in the planning process is a thorough assessment of the patient's clinical situation. The clinician must perform a comprehensive examination of the dentition and surrounding tissues in order to determine exactly what interventions are necessary.

1. **Dental condition**:
    - It is important to identify the presence of dental diseases such as tooth decay, inflammation in the gum area (periodontitis, gingivitis), and damage to the teeth (trauma, fragmentation). The condition of the teeth will determine what restoration methods can be used, including the use of fillings or crowns and bridges.
2. **Occlusion**:
    - The assessment of the contact points of the teeth and their mutual position plays a key role in diagnosis. This helps to identify possible problems such as malocclusion, missing teeth or TMJ (temporomandibular joint) dysfunction that may require intervention, both orthodontic and prosthetic.
3. **Quality of fabrics**:
    - The condition of the gums, bone and surrounding tissues must be considered to determine whether orthopaedic treatment can be successful. If the tissues are weakened or damaged, such as in cases of bone atrophy or deep gingival defects, this may require preliminary surgical interventions such as bone grafting or placement of synthetic materials to restore bone mass.

3.1.2 Defining treatment goals

The goals of prosthetic treatment can vary depending on the clinical situation, the condition of the teeth, and the overall needs of the patient. The most important goals include:

1. **Restoration of lost function**:
    - Restoring normal chewing function and improving occlusion is a priority in orthopaedic treatment. This may

include restoring lost teeth with bridges, implants or other prosthetic solutions to improve chewing and normalise jaw loading.

2. **Aesthetic Restoration**:
    - One of the most important goals of treatment is to restore the aesthetics of the dentition, especially in the smile area. This may involve the use of veneers, crowns or implants to create an attractive appearance and improve patient confidence.
3. **Elimination of painful sensations**:
    - Pain relief and discomfort associated with malocclusion, damaged teeth or TMJ dysfunction are also an important part of treatment. This may require intervention to restore teeth or correct occlusion.
4. **Prevention of further pathologies**:
    - One of the goals of dental preparation is to prevent the development of new diseases, such as gingival inflammation, periodontal disease or dental caries, which may result from improper occlusion or tooth wear. The prevention of these conditions contributes to the long-term results of prosthetic treatment.

3.1.3 Development of treatment tactics

After assessing the clinical situation and determining the treatment goals, a treatment tactic is developed, which includes the selection of an appropriate intervention method. Treatment options depend on the condition of the dentition, the presence of defects and the wishes of the patient.

1. **Conservative treatment**:

- For patients with minor dental defects, such as decay or tooth wear, conservative restoration methods may be sufficient. This includes the use of fillings, veneers or crowns to improve the function and aesthetics of the teeth.

2. **Orthodontic treatment**:
   - If it is necessary to correct the position of the teeth to normalise the occlusion, the patient may be offered orthodontic treatment. This may involve the use of braces, clear mouth guards or other orthodontic appliances to align the teeth and restore the correct bite.
3. **Orthopaedic treatment with prostheses**:
   - Dental defects such as tooth loss may require bridges, removable dentures, or implants. These treatment options restore lost teeth and normalise occlusion and chewing function.
4. **Combination treatment**:
   - In case of complex defects or occlusal disorders, a combined treatment including both orthodontic and orthopaedic methods may be proposed. This makes it possible to achieve optimal results in restoring the dentoalveolar system.

3.1.4 Predicting treatment outcome

Once a treatment plan has been developed, it is also important to predict treatment outcomes so that the patient understands what to expect during and at the end of treatment.

1. **Predicting the longevity of dentures**:
   - It is important to assess how long the fitted dentures will last. This depends on the condition of the tissue on which

they are placed and the choice of materials. Durability prediction helps to select the most suitable solutions for each individual patient.

2. **Risk Forecasting**:
    - The doctor must assess possible risks such as inflammation, infection, implant rejection or TMJ problems. This makes it possible to warn the patient of potential complications in good time and take measures to minimise them.
3. **Patient Satisfaction Assessment**:
    - It is important to predict how satisfied the patient will be with the results of treatment in terms of functionality and aesthetics. Patient expectations play an important role in the treatment process and it is important to take them into account in the planning process.

Preparing the dentition for prosthetic treatment requires a comprehensive approach that includes thorough diagnosis, assessment of the clinical situation, determination of treatment goals and selection of the best treatment tactics. The principles of planning, interdisciplinary approach and prediction of results play an important role in ensuring successful restoration of the dentoalveolar system. The harmonisation of the various treatment methods and detailed preparation allow optimal results to be achieved both functionally and aesthetically.

3.2 The role of an interdisciplinary approach

The interdisciplinary approach in orthopaedic treatment is the integration of the knowledge and expertise of specialists from different fields of medicine and dentistry, in order to achieve the best results for the patient. Orthopaedic dental treatment requires interaction with a number of other specialists, such as orthodontists, surgeons, therapists, periodontists and others, which allows for a more accurate and efficient solution to the problems associated with restoring the functionality and aesthetics of the dento-mandibular system.

3.2.1 Orthodontics and orthopaedics

One of the key areas of interdisciplinary approach in dentistry is the co-operation between orthopaedists and orthodontists. Although both specialists work within the framework of restoring dental functionality, their tasks are different and successful treatment often requires a coordinated approach.

- **The role of an orthodontist** is to correct the position of teeth, correct bite irregularities and prepare the teeth for orthopaedic appliances. Orthodontists diagnose and correct abnormalities such as crowding and misalignment of the teeth and create the conditions for future orthopaedic interventions such as implants and bridges. The correct positioning of the teeth is important to avoid stress on the TMJ and teeth and to ensure the stability and durability of the dentures.
- **The role of the orthodontist** is to restore lost teeth and ensure the overall functionality of the masticatory system. The orthopaedist must take into account the changes caused by orthodontic treatment, such as improved occlusion or alignment of the tooth rows, in order to correctly develop a strategy for the placement of the final prosthetic structures (crowns, implants or bridges). It is important that the orthodontist takes into account the degree of stabilisation of the tooth rows after orthodontic treatment , which affects the further loading of the teeth and gums.

The coordinated interaction between the orthodontist and prosthodontist helps provide a comprehensive approach to addressing bite problems and restoring lost teeth, which helps to achieve long-lasting, high-quality results.

3.2.2 Surgery and prosthetics

In some cases, surgeons may be required to successfully prepare the teeth for dentures, implants or other prosthetic devices. Surgical intervention required to restore the dentoalveolar system may include the following procedures:

1. **Tooth** extraction: Tooth extraction often becomes necessary when teeth are severely damaged, cannot be repaired, or are a source of infection or other complications. Tooth extraction may be part of the preparation for implants or to create space for other prosthetic structures such as bridges.
2. **Gingivoplasty**: Gingivoplasty is a plastic surgery on the gum, aimed at correcting its shape to create optimal conditions for the placement of implants, crowns or other prostheses. This method helps to improve the aesthetic appearance and prevent future pathological changes in the gums.
3. **Bone** grafting: If there is insufficient bone tissue for implants, bone grafting is necessary. This surgical procedure aims to restore bone volume and density for successful implantation. Bone grafting options include:
    - **A sinus lift** is a procedure to raise the bone level in the upper jaw area, necessary when there is insufficient bone height to accommodate implants.

- **Bone grafts** - the use of the patient's bone tissue or synthetic materials to restore the necessary bone volume to facilitate successful implantation.

Thus, surgical intervention plays an important role in preparing the dentition for the placement of prosthetic structures, especially in cases of bone deficiency or damage to the teeth and gums.

3.2.3 Therapist and periodontist

Therapists and periodontists fulfil a key role in the initial stages of preparing the dentition for prosthetic treatment, as they treat tooth and gum disease, which directly affects the choice and effectiveness of further prosthetic interventions.

1. **Therapist**: The therapist treats tooth decay, pulpitis and other dental diseases that may affect the possibility of fitting dentures. By treating tooth decay and eliminating infectious foci, the conditions for the safe and durable fitting of prosthetic devices can be created. For example, it is important to remove all carious lesions from the teeth before starting the placement of crowns or implants.
2. **Periodontist**: Periodontists specialise in gum diseases such as periodontitis and gingivitis. Treating these conditions is critical to preparing the teeth, as healthy gums and periodontal tissues are the foundation for dentures. Periodontists treat inflammation, repair tissue and strengthen teeth, which prevents possible complications when implants or other structures are placed.

3.3 Surgical preparation methods

In some cases, teeth require surgical preparation prior to the placement of dentures, implants, or other prosthetic devices. Surgery may be necessary in cases of severe defects in the bone, teeth or gums, and it plays a key role in ensuring the stability and longevity of prosthetic solutions.

3.3.1 Removal of teeth

Tooth extraction is one of the most common surgical procedures in dental preparation. This procedure is necessary when teeth are severely decayed or cannot be repaired, as well as when there is inflammation that can lead to complications. Tooth extraction may also be necessary to create space for implants or other dentures.

3.3.2 Gingival surgery

Gum surgeries may be necessary to create optimal conditions for the placement of prosthetic structures such as implants, bridges or crowns. These surgeries include:

- **Gingivoplasty** - improving the aesthetics of the gums and preparing them for the installation of orthopaedic structures.
- A gingenectomy is the removal of part of the gum to improve access to or appearance of teeth.
- **Gum repositioning** - moving the gum to improve its position, which helps to protect the roots of the teeth and prevent inflammation.

3.3.3 Bone grafting

Bone grafting is necessary when there is not enough bone tissue to accommodate implants. This may be due to bone atrophy or insufficient bone thickness and height. Bone grafting includes the following types of surgery:

- **A sinus lift** is a surgery designed to increase the level of bone in the upper jaw to create the conditions for successful implantation.
- **Bone grafts** are the use of a patient's bone tissue or synthetic materials to restore the amount of bone needed for implantation.

These procedures create the right bone structure for the placement of implants and other structures, which contributes to the longevity and functionality of the teeth.

Conclusion

Thus, preparation of the dentition for orthopaedic treatment requires a comprehensive approach involving interdisciplinary cooperation of specialists from different fields of medicine and dentistry. The success of treatment largely depends on the coordination of orthopaedist, orthodontist, surgeon, therapist and periodontist. The use of surgical methods such as tooth extraction, gum surgery and bone grafting, as well as professional co-operation between specialists, allows for the longevity and high functionality of prostheses and implants.

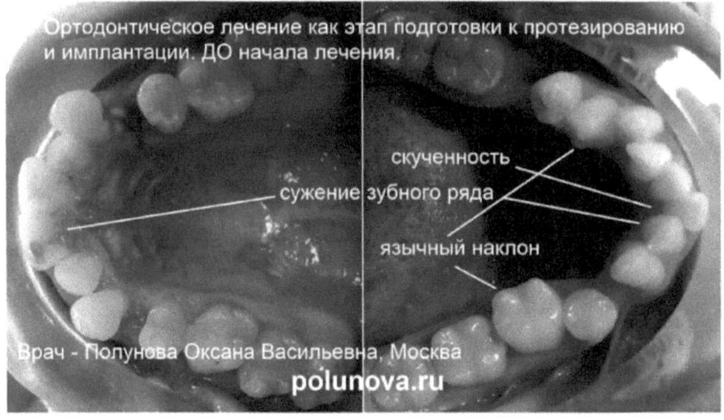

Chapter 4. Treatment of secondary deformities

The treatment of secondary deformities of the dentoalveolar system is a complex and multifaceted process that involves various techniques aimed at restoring normal function and aesthetics of the teeth. These deformities can be the result of trauma, disease, growth disorders or heredity and require an individualised approach. The main treatment modalities are orthodontic treatment, prosthodontics and implantology. In some cases, treatment may involve a combined approach, using several methods depending on the degree and nature of the deformity.

4.1 Orthodontic treatment

Orthodontic treatment of secondary deformities of the dentoalveolar system is the most important stage aimed at correcting anomalies of the dental rows and bite. Orthodontics allows not only to restore the functionality of the chewing apparatus, but also to significantly improve aesthetic indicators, which is important for patients seeking to restore the normal appearance of teeth.

4.1.1 Principles of orthodontic treatment

Orthodontic treatment is aimed at correcting anomalies such as malposition of teeth, imbalances in the ratio of the upper and lower jaw, and developmental anomalies of the temporomandibular joint (TMJ). It is important that treatment is comprehensive and consistent, taking into account all the patient's characteristics.

1. **Diagnosis and planning**: The basis for successful orthodontic treatment is a thorough diagnosis and treatment plan. At this stage,

the orthodontist performs a comprehensive examination of the patient, including:

- Assessment of the condition of the teeth and gums.
- An occlusion analysis, which is the study of how the teeth of the upper and lower jaw touch each other.
- Identification of factors that may have influenced the development of the deformity (injuries, diseases, growth disorders, genetic factors, etc.).

Taking into account the findings, an individualised treatment plan is developed, which determines the sequence of steps and suitable correction methods.

2. **Use of different appliances**: Depending on the clinical situation and the degree of deformity, different types of orthodontic appliances can be used:
   - **Braces** are the most common devices for correcting the position of teeth. Modern braces (metal, ceramic, sapphire) can effectively correct even complex deformities such as crowding, open bite, deep bite and others.
   - **Trainers and mouthguards** - used to correct minor anomalies or as auxiliary appliances, e.g. in the preparatory period before more complex procedures.
   - **Myofunctional appliances** - used to treat deformities caused by muscle dysfunction (e.g. finger sucking habits or mouth breathing disorders), which can affect the position of the teeth and jaws.
3. **Stages of orthodontic** treatment: Orthodontic treatment can be divided into several successive stages:
   - **Preparatory phase**: includes treatment of dental diseases (tooth decay, gum inflammation), strengthening of the teeth

and restoration of their functionality. This stage is important to ensure the success of further treatment.

  - **Main** stage: at this stage, orthodontic appliances (braces, mouth guards and others) are fitted to correct the position of the teeth and normalise the occlusion.
  - **The final stage**: includes consolidation of the achieved results with the help of retainers - special appliances that help to maintain the correct position of the teeth after the braces are removed.

4. **Combined** treatment: In some cases, orthodontic treatment is combined with other methods such as surgery or prosthetics. This may be necessary to achieve the best possible result, especially in complex cases such as jaw growth abnormalities or severe deformities.

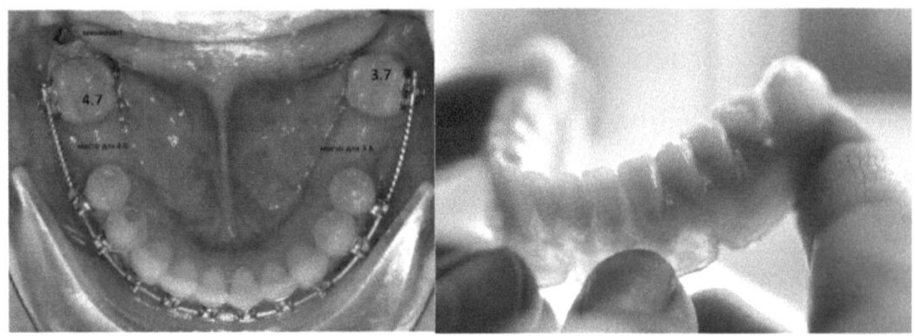

4.1.2 Indications and contraindications

Orthodontic treatment is indicated in the presence of various disorders of the dentoalveolar system:

1. **Indications**:
  - Bite disorders such as distal, mesial, open, crossbite.
  - The crowding or excessive spacing of teeth.
  - Developmental anomalies of the TMJ.

- Jaw growth disorders (e.g., hypoplasia of the upper or lower jaw).
- Some cases of TMJ dysfunction associated with misaligned teeth or jaws.

2. **Contraindications**: Orthodontic treatment has a number of contraindications, including:
   - Severe gum or dental disease that requires prior treatment (e.g. periodontitis, tooth decay, pulpitis).
   - Conditions for which braces cannot be used (e.g. osteoporosis or other bone diseases that may affect the outcome of treatment).
   - Patients with developmental disorders that require surgical intervention, such as significant jaw deformities that cannot be corrected by orthodontic methods alone.

4.1.3 Benefits of orthodontic treatment

Orthodontic treatment for secondary deformities has many advantages:

- **Restoration of function**: correct occlusion can normalise chewing function, improve diction and prevent temporomandibular joint disorders.
- **Aesthetic improvement**: correction of dental and bite deformities improves the patient's appearance, which plays an important role in social adaptation and confidence.
- **Prevention of further diseases**: correcting an incorrect bite and positioning of the teeth helps to prevent the development of tooth and gum diseases such as tooth decay and periodontitis and reduces the strain on the TMJ.

Orthodontic treatment is an integral part of a comprehensive rehabilitation programme for the dento-alveolar system, helping to improve both the functionality and aesthetics of the teeth.

4.2 Prosthetics (removable and fixed)

Dentures are an essential part of the comprehensive treatment of secondary deformities of the dentoalveolar system, especially in cases of significant damage to or loss of teeth. Dentures can restore chewing function, improve aesthetics and provide the patient with comfort in everyday life. Depending on the condition of the teeth, the patient's clinical situation and their preferences, dentures can be removable or fixed. The choice between them depends on many factors, including jaw anatomy, financial possibilities and the patient's wishes.

4.2.1 Removable dentures

Removable dentures are structures that can be removed by the patient for maintenance and cleaning as well as for routine check-ups with the dentist. They are used in cases where fixed dentures cannot be fitted, e.g. in cases of significant tooth loss or missing teeth on one or both jaws.

Advantages of removable dentures:

- **Affordability**: Removable dentures are often less expensive than fixed dentures, making them more accessible to patients on a tight budget.
- **Ease of fabrication**: These dentures are easier to fabricate and the fitting process usually takes less time.
- **Versatility**: Removable dentures can be used in cases where fixed prostheses are not possible, e.g. when teeth are missing in several areas of the jaw.

- **Easy care**: The patient can remove the denture for regular maintenance, cleaning and prevention of gum disease.

Disadvantages of removable dentures:

- **Discomfort**: Removable dentures can be uncomfortable to wear, especially at first. Patients often complain of incomplete stability and a foreign body sensation in the mouth.
- **Need for** adjustments: Due to changes in the structure of the teeth or gums, removable dentures require regular adjustments and replacements.
- **Psychological aspect**: Patients may feel insecure about the appearance of removable dentures, especially if they are visible when talking or laughing.

Types of removable dentures:

1. **Complete removable dentures** - used when there is a complete absence of teeth in both jaws. These dentures replace the entire tooth row and can be made of different materials such as acrylic or nylon components.
2. **Partial removable dentures** - used to restore one or more lost teeth. They can be made with metal frameworks for added strength and reliability

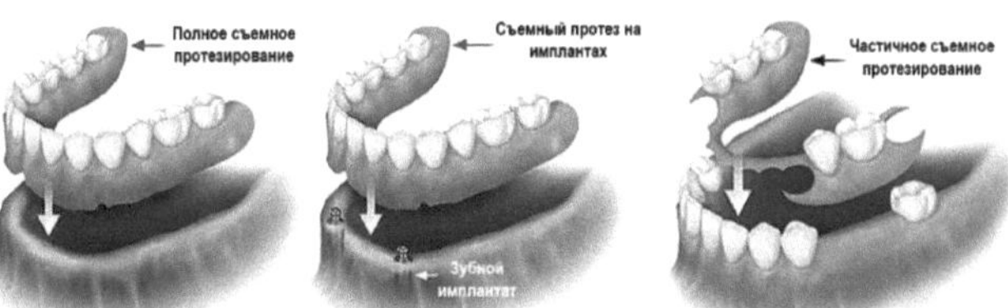

4.2.2 Fixed dentures

Fixed dentures are permanently fitted and cannot be removed by the patient. They provide greater stability, comfort and aesthetic appeal, making them the preferred choice for most patients. Fixed dentures include crowns, bridges and implant-supported dentures.

Advantages of fixed dentures:

- **High stability**: Fixed dentures are securely anchored and do not require additional effort for insertion or adjustment. They are more stable, which reduces the risk of them falling out.
- **Comfort**: Patients generally experience less discomfort with fixed dentures because they feel like natural teeth.
- **Aesthetic effect**: Modern materials for fixed dentures (e.g. ceramics) make it possible to create designs that mimic natural teeth as closely as possible, both in shape and colour.
- **Durability**: Fixed dentures have a long lifespan and can last for decades with proper care.

Несъемное протезирование

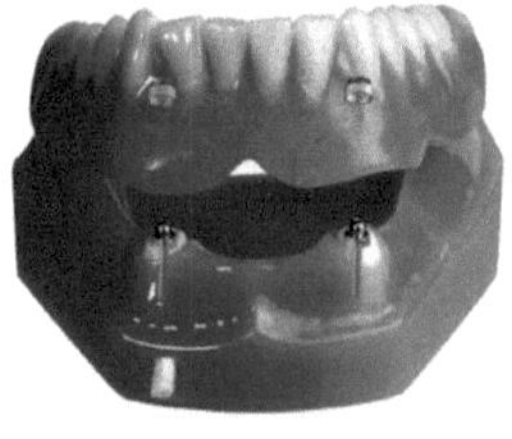

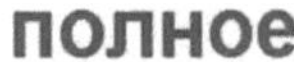

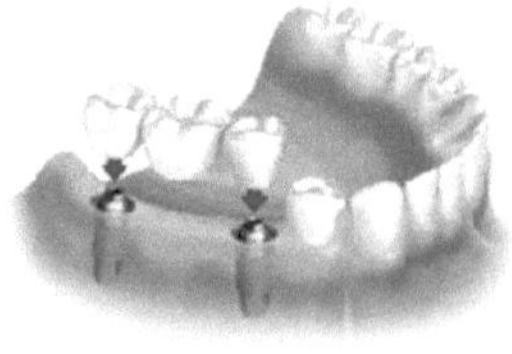

Types of fixed dentures:

1. **Crowns** are dentures that cover the entire tooth, restoring its shape, size, and function. Crowns can be metal, ceramic, or a

combination. They are used for significant tooth damage, such as tooth decay due to decay or trauma.

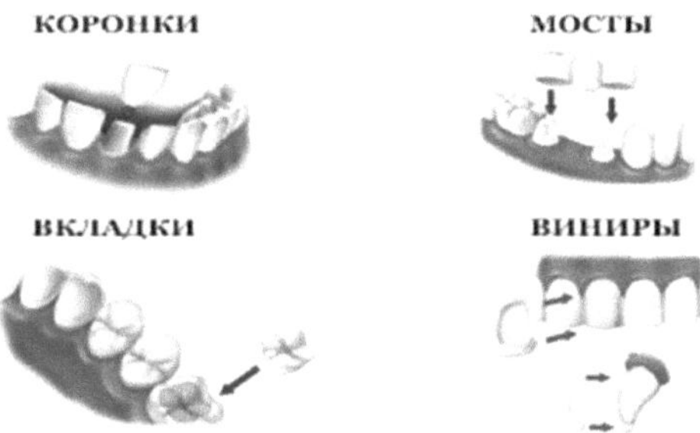

2. **Bridges** - used to restore several lost teeth. The denture consists of artificial teeth that are placed on top of the remaining healthy teeth, thus creating a bridge.
3. **Implant** dentures are **prostheses** fitted on dental implants that are implanted into the jaw. This method is particularly suitable for restoring teeth if natural teeth have been completely lost.

ВИДЫ СЪЁМНОГО ПРОТЕЗИРОВАНИЯ
с опорой на дентальные имплантаты

съемный протез с фиксацией к специальным замкам, установленным на имплантаты

съемный протез с опорой на балку (или балки), установленную на имплантаты

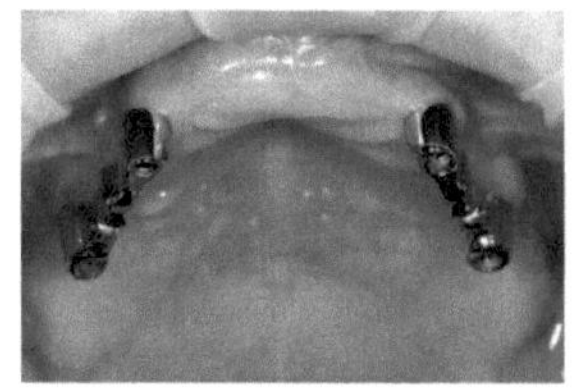

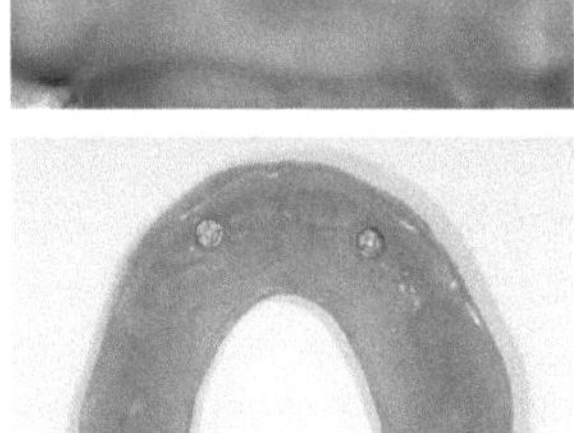

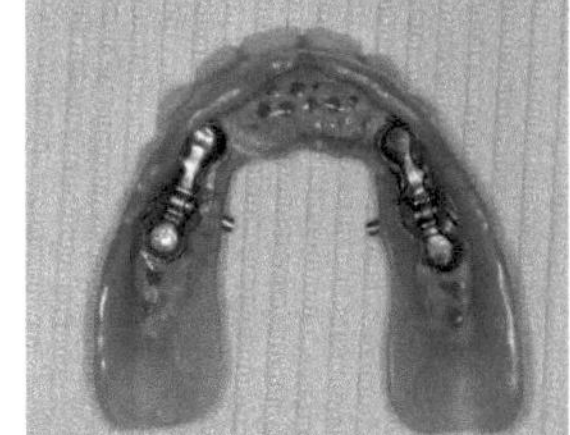

4.2.3 Planning and stages of prosthetic treatment

The process of dentures is a multi-step procedure that includes diagnosis, preparation of the teeth, fabrication of the dentures and their placement. The success of dentures depends on careful planning and execution of all the steps.

1. **Diagnosis and assessment of the condition of the teeth**: The first stage involves a comprehensive diagnosis, including an examination of the teeth, gums and x-rays. This helps to determine the extent of tooth loss, bone and gum health, as well as the possibility of using certain prosthetic methods.
2. **Preparing** the teeth: If the teeth need to be ground (e.g. for crowns) in order to fit the denture, they are prepared at this stage. In some cases, tooth or gum diseases such as tooth decay, gum inflammation or periodontitis need to be treated.
3. **Impressions and fabrication of dentures**: After preparing the teeth, the specialist takes impressions of the patient's teeth, which are used to create individual dentures. Depending on the type of denture, different materials are used, such as acrylic, metal, ceramics, and composites.
4. **Denture placement and correction**: At this stage, the dentures are placed on the teeth and their fit and comfort for the patient are checked. Once the dentures are in place, additional adjustments may be required to achieve optimal bite, aesthetics, and comfort. It is important that the dentures fit perfectly and do not cause discomfort when chewing or talking.

Dentures are therefore an important part of the restoration of the maxillofacial system, allowing patients to regain lost dental function and aesthetic appearance. The correct choice of the type of prosthesis, careful planning and quality execution of all stages of prosthetics are the key to a successful and long-lasting result.

4.3 Implantology as part of a holistic approach

Implantology is an essential component of a comprehensive approach in the treatment of secondary deformities of the dento-mandibular system, especially in cases of tooth loss. Dental implants are artificial roots that are placed in the jawbone to replace lost teeth. This method makes it possible to restore not only the aesthetics but also the functionality of the dento-mandibular system with minimal intervention and a high degree of longevity.

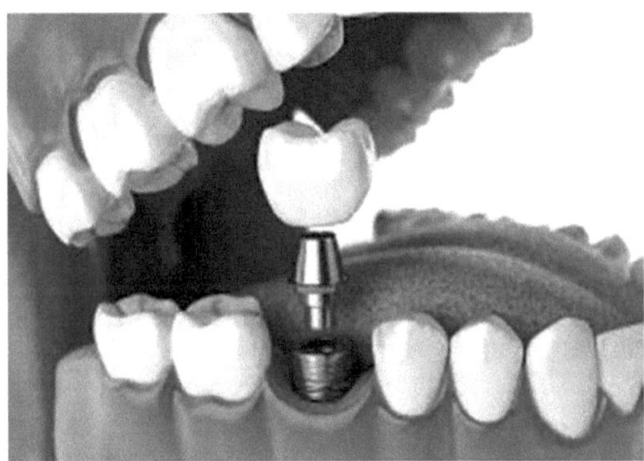

4.3.1 Benefits of implantology

1. **Bone preservation**: Dental implants help to prevent bone loss that inevitably occurs with long-term tooth loss. The implant stimulates the bone tissue to maintain its volume, which is especially important in the complete absence of teeth. This avoids the need for complex bone restoration procedures (e.g. bone grafting).
2. **Stability and longevity**: Dental implants, properly placed and cared for, can last for decades, providing high functionality and

comfort for the patient. Unlike removable dentures, which require regular adjustments and may be less stable, implants provide stability and longevity.

3. **Aesthetic advantages**: Modern dental implants can be fitted with ceramic or zirconia crowns that fully mimic natural teeth. This allows for excellent aesthetic results that are as good as the appearance of natural teeth. The implants can be perfectly matched in colour and shape, which is especially important for patients who care about their appearance.
4. **Functional support**: In addition to aesthetic benefits, implants restore normal chewing function, allowing patients to chew their food fully again. This improves quality of life and promotes proper digestion, as it restores the load on the jawbone and promotes its health.
5. **Minimising damage to neighbouring** teeth: Unlike bridges, which require the grinding of neighbouring teeth to fit them, implants do not involve healthy teeth, minimising the risk of damage to them.

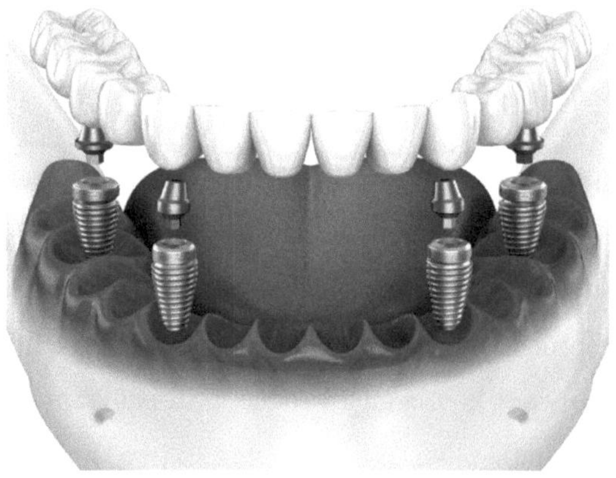

4.3.2 Implant placement process

The process of dental implant placement involves several key steps, each of which requires a highly qualified specialist.

1. **Patient assessment**: Before implants are placed, a thorough diagnostic evaluation, including radiographs and computed tomography (CT) scans, must be performed to assess bone health and identify possible contraindications. It is also important to determine the type of implant that will be most effective for your particular case.
2. **Surgical** stage: In this stage, the implant is implanted into the jawbone. The surgery is performed under local anaesthesia and usually takes between 30 minutes and several hours, depending on the complexity of the case. It is important that the surgeon uses modern technology (e.g. 3D planning) to accurately place the implant in the bone, which increases the likelihood of successful integration of the implant.
3. **Recovery phase**: After implant placement, there is a healing period that can last from 3 to 6 months. During this period, the implant fuses with the bone tissue, a process known as osseointegration. It is important that the patient follows the doctor's recommendations during this period to avoid infections and other complications.
4. **Implant prosthesis placement**: After successful fusion of the implant with the bone tissue, a prosthesis (crown, bridge or removable prosthesis) is placed. The prosthesis is customised to the patient's anatomy to ensure comfort and a natural appearance.

4.3.3 Application of implantology in secondary deformities

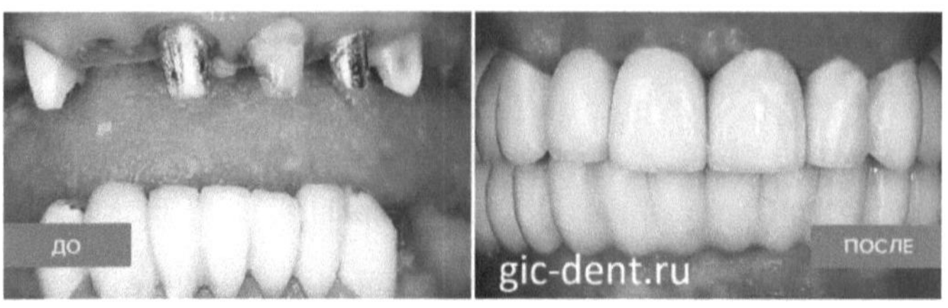

Implantology plays a key role in the treatment of secondary deformities, especially in cases where tooth loss leads to functional and aesthetic problems. In such cases, implants are used to restore lost teeth and ensure a correct bite.

- **Restoration of lost teeth**: If one or more teeth are lost, implants can be placed to restore the tooth row. This avoids deformation of adjacent teeth and loss of chewing function.
- **Implant-supported** bridges: If several teeth are lost, implants can be used for the placement of bridges, which offer stability and durability compared to traditional removable structures.
- Implant **prostheses for patients with deformities**: Implantology is particularly important for patients with deformities caused by trauma, gum disease, jaw growth abnormalities or even congenital defects. In such cases, implants can restore the normal position of the teeth and jaws, improving both aesthetic and functional results.
- **Treatment of gum disease and its consequences**: Implant placement can also be used to restore teeth in patients with chronic gum disease such as periodontitis. In such cases, implantology can be a better alternative to traditional prosthetic methods, as implants can stimulate the bone and prevent further atrophy.
- **Use in complex treatment**: Implantology is often combined with orthodontic treatment and prosthetics. For example, after bite correction with orthodontic appliances, implants can be placed to

restore lost teeth, improving not only the functional but also the aesthetic characteristics of the maxillofacial system.

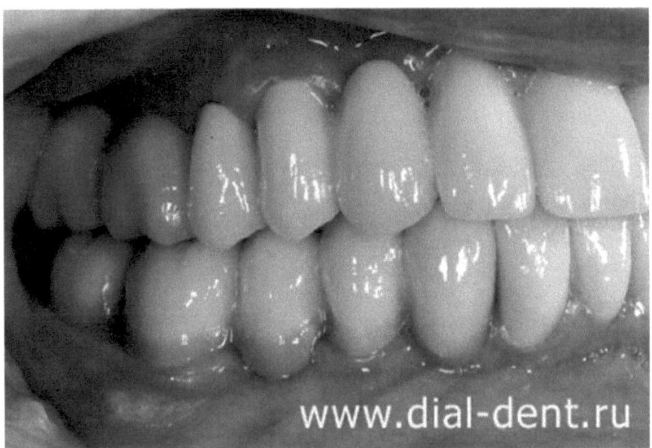

Thus, implantology is an important component in the treatment of secondary deformities of the dento-mandibular system, providing long-term and highly effective results. A comprehensive approach, including implantological, orthodontic and prosthetic methods, allows patients to regain lost function, restore the aesthetic appearance of teeth and improve their quality of life.

Chapter 5. Rehabilitation of patients

Rehabilitation of patients after orthopaedic and orthodontic treatment of secondary deformities of the dentoalveolar system is a crucial stage aimed at full restoration of both physical function and psychological comfort of the patient. It includes several key components: psychological support, supportive treatment and prophylaxis, and regular analyses of long-term results, which allow the effectiveness of the treatment performed to be evaluated and possible complications to be prevented. These aspects are important for achieving a sustainable and long-term result, both functionally and aesthetically.

5.1 Psychological aspects of rehabilitation

Psychological support plays a key role in the rehabilitation process, especially after orthopaedic treatment and the fitting of complex prostheses or implants. Dental disorders can have a significant impact on the patient's self-esteem, self-confidence and social adaptation. Psychological discomfort caused by external defects can slow down the healing process if the patient's emotional and psychological needs are not addressed. The importance of psychological support at all stages of treatment and rehabilitation can hardly be overestimated, as it contributes not only to successful recovery, but also to the formation of sustainable, positive results.

5.1.1 Impact of deformities on the psycho-emotional state of the patient

Maxillofacial deformities, especially those that require the intervention of an orthopaedist or orthodontist, can have a significant impact on patients' perception of their appearance. Changes in the bite, loss of teeth or defects in their position often cause the following psycho-emotional problems:

1. **Psychological discomfort**: Patients with jaw deformities often feel embarrassed or ashamed of the appearance of their teeth. This can lead to decreased self-confidence, feelings of inferiority, and even social isolation. Patients may avoid socialising, feel embarrassed to smile, which exacerbates the problems and causes further difficulties in personal and professional relationships.
2. **Social anxiety**: Patients with dental deformities often worry about not being able to communicate or smile freely, fearing how they are perceived by others. This can cause anxiety in social situations, where a person worries about being judged or rejected because of their appearance. This can lead to limited social contact and a reduced quality of life.
3. **Depression and stress**: Often patients suffering from dental disease or tooth loss experience stress, depression or anxiety disorders. These emotional states can make the rehabilitation process much more difficult. Psychological stress increases the physical discomfort associated with treatment and can make it difficult to adjust to new dentures or implants. This emphasises the importance of the intervention of a psychologist or psychotherapist in the comprehensive rehabilitation of patients.
4. **Psychological barriers to treatment**: Patients who are worried about external deformities may delay the start of treatment or avoid treatment due to fear of pain, the length of the process or lack of confidence in the treatment methods. This can delay or complicate the rehabilitation process itself.

5.1.2 Psychological support and correction methods

Psychological support is an integral part of rehabilitation and should address several important aspects:

1. **Reducing stress and anxiety**: It is important that patients feel confident and comfortable during and after treatment. Relaxation techniques such as breathing exercises, yoga or meditation may be used to help patients reduce stress and tension. Psychotherapy sessions can help patients overcome fears related to treatment and rehabilitation.
2. **Psychological counselling**: Working with a psychologist helps patients to cope with low self-esteem and emotional difficulties associated with dentoalveolar deformities. The specialist may use cognitive behavioural therapy (CBT), which aims to change negative thoughts and beliefs, increase self-confidence and acceptance of one's appearance.
3. **Group sessions and support**: Support programmes that include meeting other patients experiencing similar problems can be helpful. Peer support and sharing experiences can help patients feel that they are not alone and can increase motivation to continue treatment and recovery.
4. **Education programmes**: Educating patients about the treatment process and possible outcomes also helps to reduce anxiety. Knowing how treatment will proceed and what to expect at each stage can significantly reduce psychological distress.
5. **Psychological adjustment to new dentures or implants**: Dentures or implants that have been placed take time to get used to. Patients may feel discomfort or aversion to the new structures. At such times, psychological support is important to help the patient adapt and accept the prosthesis or implant as a natural part of their body.

5.1.3 Impact of successful rehabilitation on the psycho-emotional state of the patient

Properly organised rehabilitation and successful restoration of the dento-mandibular system, both functionally and aesthetically, have a profound effect on the psycho-emotional state of the patient. When patients see positive changes in their appearance, when chewing function is restored and speech problems disappear, their self-confidence increases significantly.

- **Enhanced social adaptation**: After successful treatment, patients often return to a normal social life and become more confident in socialising without being self-conscious about their appearance. This can significantly improve their quality of life and reduce their stress levels.
- **Improved psychological well-being**: Restoring normal aesthetics and function of the maxillofacial system helps patients relieve feelings of shame and depression, improving their self-esteem and overall psychological **well-being**.
- **Increased motivation to maintain results**: After a successful restoration, it is easier for patients to monitor the condition of their teeth and follow the doctor's recommendations for preventive care, which also contributes to a long-lasting treatment result.

Thus, an integrated approach to patient rehabilitation includes not only physiological recovery, but also psychological support, which ensures higher treatment efficiency and contributes to the patient's successful adaptation to society.

5.1.2 The role of the psychologist in the rehabilitation process

Psychological support for the patient during rehabilitation is an important element in achieving a positive outcome. A psychologist can help the patient:

- **Overcome fear and anxiety**: Often patients are anxious about upcoming surgical procedures, such as implants. A psychologist can work with the patient to reduce stress and fear by educating them about the treatment and its safety.
- **Strengthen motivation**: The treatment process can be long and require patience. A psychologist helps the patient to stay motivated and supports them through difficult moments.
- **Work with self-esteem**: The psychologist helps the patient to improve self-perception, deal with complexes related to appearance and maintain a positive attitude towards treatment.

5.1.3 Social adaptation

Special attention in rehabilitation should be paid to the patient's social adaptation. In some cases, the restoration of the maxillary system allows the patient to return to a normal social life, improve their ability to communicate with others and restore lost social ties. It is also important to work with the patient's loved ones to ensure that they support the patient during the rehabilitation process and understand their concerns.

5.2 Supportive treatment and prevention

Supportive treatment and prevention play a key role in the long-term success of orthopaedic and orthodontic treatment, ensuring sustainable and long-lasting results after the active phase of therapy is complete. Even after deformities have been corrected and the maxillofacial system has been restored, it is important to adhere to the recommendations of the specialists at to prevent relapses, maintain the health of the teeth and gums, and ensure the longevity of the fitted prostheses and implants. Preventive measures not only help to maintain the results of treatment, but also to prevent the emergence of new dental diseases.

5.2.1 Supportive treatment

Maintenance treatment includes measures aimed at maintaining the health of the maxillofacial system, stabilising the achieved results and preventing possible complications. The main components of maintenance treatment:

1. **Regular check-ups**: After the main stage of treatment has been completed, the patient should have regular check-ups with a dentist or prosthodontist. This is necessary to monitor the condition of the teeth, gums, as well as to check that the dentures and implants are fitted correctly. Timely detection of possible problems helps to avoid complications and prolong the service life of the installed structures.
2. **Denture** adjustments: In the first few months after the placement of dentures or implants, the patient may experience discomfort or feel the need for minor adjustments. These adjustments may include reshaping the dentures, fixing them, or adapting the implants to help improve comfort and functionality. Particular attention should be paid to adjustments in the first year after placement, when the oral tissues are still adapting to the changes.
3. **Oral** care: Patients are provided with oral care recommendations to prevent gum disease or tooth decay, as well as care for implants and dentures. This includes proper brushing techniques, flossing, and the use of antiseptic rinses to help maintain healthy gums and prevent inflammation.

4. **Preventive check-ups with allied specialists**: In some cases, it may be necessary to consult with other specialists, such as a periodontist, if the patient has a tendency to have gum disease. Systematic bite and jaw checks with an orthodontist may also be part of maintenance treatment.

5.2.2 Disease prevention

Preventive measures play a key role in maintaining long-term dental health. Proper disease prevention can prevent the development of complications and ensure the long-term survival of treatment results:

1. **Gum** disease **prevention**: Gum disease, such as periodontitis and gingivitis, can cause tooth loss or affect the stability of implants. To prevent these diseases, regular hygienic cleanings at the dentist, the use of antibacterial rinses and toothpastes, and maintaining good hygiene at home are recommended. It is especially important to look after the condition of the gums where dentures and implants are placed, where inflammation often occurs.
2. **Caries** prevention: To prevent tooth decay, it is important to practice good oral hygiene, including brushing twice a day with toothpaste containing fluoride. It is also important to limit sugar intake, especially in the form of sugary drinks and foods that can be a source of bacterial activity in the mouth. Regular professional cleanings at the dentist are also important to prevent tooth decay and gum disease.
3. **Use of retainers**: After orthodontic treatment, the use of retainers (plates or mouth guards) is an important preventive measure to maintain the correct position of the teeth. Retainers prevent the recurrence of deformities and help to consolidate the results of

treatment. It is important that the patient adheres to the doctor's recommendations regarding the timing and wearing regime of the retainers.

4. **Monitoring the health of implants and dentures**: Patients who use implants or dentures should have them checked regularly to make sure there is no tissue inflammation, infection, or other problems. Supporting the maxillofacial system with regular checkups and implant care can help avoid problems such as peri-implantitis (inflammation of the tissue around the implant).

5.2.3 Lifestyle and diet

A patient's lifestyle and nutrition play an important role in preventing diseases of the dentoalveolar system and maintaining its health. A few key recommendations:

1. **Avoiding bad habits**: Smoking, excessive alcohol consumption, and habits such as teeth grinding (bruxism) or chewing hard objects (pencils, fingernails) can negatively affect the condition of teeth, gums and implants. Smoking in particular is associated with an increased risk of gum disease, a weakened immune system and reduced tissue healing ability.
2. **Good nutrition**: A diet rich in vitamins, minerals and calcium helps to strengthen tooth enamel and maintain healthy gums and bones. It is advisable to include foods containing phosphorus, vitamins A, D, E and foods rich in antioxidants such as vegetables, fruits and nuts in the diet. It is important to avoid excessive consumption of sugar and carbohydrates to prevent tooth decay and gum disease.
3. **Regular physical** activity: Maintaining physical activity helps to improve blood circulation, which has a positive effect on the

health of the oral tissues. Physical activity also helps to reduce stress and improve overall body health, which helps the body to recover faster from procedures and maintain normal immune system function.

4. **Limit chewing** hard foods: Chewing excessively hard foods such as nuts, ice or pips can cause damage to teeth, dentures or implants. Patients should avoid these habits to prevent damage and ensure the longevity of the implants.

5.2.4 Monitoring and long-term results

One of the most important aspects of maintenance treatment is regular monitoring of the long-term results of treatment. Systematic follow-up helps to identify possible problems at an early stage, to correct therapeutic actions in time and to prevent the development of complications. It is important that the patient continues to co-operate with the doctor and adheres to the recommendations in order to maintain and improve the achieved results.

5.3 Analysing long-term results

Analysing long-term results is an important stage in the rehabilitation of patients, as it allows not only to assess the success of the treatment, but also to identify possible complications that may arise in the future.

5.3.1 Evaluating the effectiveness of treatment

Various methods are used to assess the long-term effectiveness of treatment:

- **Functional outcome assessment**: This includes checking chewing function, assessing the stability of dentures or implants, and analysing TMJ function.

- **Aesthetic assessment**: An important aspect is the restoration of the aesthetics of the dentition, i.e. to what extent the teeth have been successfully restored in terms of appearance and to what extent the patient is satisfied with this.

5.3.2 Identifying complications

Even with successful treatment, complications can occur, such as:

- **Implant rejection**: In rare cases, implants may fail to take root, requiring additional interventions.
- **Gum problems**: Infections or inflammation of the gums around implants or dentures can occur if oral care recommendations are not followed.
- **Denture wear or damage**: Dentures may need to be replaced or adjusted due to wear and tear, which may result in the need for re-intervention.

5.3.3 Durability of treatment

The longevity of treatment results depends on many factors, such as proper care of the teeth and dentures, adherence to the dentist's recommendations, and the absence of diseases affecting the dento-mandibular system. Ideally, treatment results should last for many years if all recommendations are followed.

5.3.4 Patient satisfaction

One of the key indicators of treatment success is patient satisfaction with the results. This is assessed through surveys, interviews and patient observation. It is important that the patient feels comfortable and confident in their new dentoalveolar system, which directly affects their quality of life.

Thus, rehabilitation of patients after orthopaedic and orthodontic treatment of secondary deformities includes not only physical restoration of the dentoalveolar system, but also support at the psychological level. Supportive treatment and prophylaxis help to maintain the results of treatment, and regular analyses of long-term results allow for timely identification of possible problems and prevention of complications.

Conclusion

The treatment of secondary deformities of the dentoalveolar system is a complex and multifaceted process that requires a comprehensive approach. Accurate diagnosis, individually tailored orthodontic and prosthetic treatment, and the use of modern technologies such as implantology and 3D modelling are important components of this process. However, the success of treatment is not limited to the physical restoration of the maxillary system, but also includes the psychological rehabilitation of the patient, supportive treatment and prevention, and long-term evaluation of the results.

During rehabilitation, it is important to consider not only the physical aspects, but also the psychological aspects. Patients who are worried about external defects or functional problems require appropriate psychological support, which plays a key role in successfully restoring their confidence and social adaptation. Supportive treatment and prevention are also essential for the longevity of treatment results, preventing recurrences and maintaining the health of the maxillofacial system for many years.

Key Findings:

1. **Comprehensive Approach**: Treatment of secondary malocclusion requires a comprehensive approach that combines orthodontic, orthopaedic and implantology techniques. Each of these methods plays its unique role in restoring normal function and aesthetics to the dentoalveolar system.
2. **The importance of psychological support**: Psychological aspects of treatment are important because a malocclusion or tooth loss can significantly affect the patient's self-esteem. Psychological

support and working with the patient on their self-perception are important elements of successful rehabilitation.

3. **Supportive treatment and prevention**: After completion of the main phase of treatment, regular check-ups, preventive measures and oral care recommendations should be carried out to prevent complications and maintain long-term results.
4. **Long-term effectiveness of treatment**: Regular analyses of long-term results help to identify possible problems at an early stage and assess the effectiveness of the treatment in terms of functional and aesthetic results.

Recommendations for clinical practice:

1. **Integration of different treatment methods**: It is important to combine orthodontic and prosthetic treatment with implantological interventions to obtain the most sustainable and effective result. The use of 3D modelling and other modern technologies will help to improve the accuracy of diagnosis and treatment planning.
2. **Psychological support for patients**: Every patient should receive psychological support throughout the treatment process, including information about upcoming treatment and possible consequences. Psychological preparation helps to avoid patient stress and anxiety.
3. **Regular monitoring and prevention**: After completion of the main treatment, it is important to advise patients to have regular follow-up examinations, use of retainers, and prevention of gum disease and caries to maintain treatment results and avoid recurrences.
4. **Patient education on oral care**: Patients should be educated on the proper care of teeth and dentures, including the use of special

hygiene products and prophylactic rinses to prevent gum disease and tooth decay.

5. **Long-term evaluation of results**: It is important not only to record the current results of treatment, but also to conduct a long-term evaluation of the maxillofacial system in order to intervene in time if complications or new problems arise.

Thus, successful treatment of secondary deformities requires the coordinated work of specialists from various fields of medicine and dentistry, as well as consideration of all factors affecting the patient's health. A combined approach including diagnosis, treatment and rehabilitation can maximise the results in restoring the health of the dento-mandibular system and improving the patient's quality of life.

List of references

1. **Kuzmin, V. A.** (2018). *Modern methods of diagnostics and treatment of diseases of the dentoalveolar system.* Moscow: Medical Book.
2. **Petrova, I. A.** (2017). *Fundamentals of orthodontics and orthopaedics: theory and practice*. SPb.: Nauchnaya Mysl.
3. **Galkin, M. V.** (2019). *Implantology in the complex treatment of diseases of the dento-mandibular system*. Moscow: SpetsLit.
4. **Dmitrieva, S. V.** (2020). *Orthopaedic treatment of secondary deformities of the dentoalveolar system*. Moscow: Rudomino.
5. **Efremova, I. I.** (2017). *Rehabilitation of patients with diseases of the dentoalveolar system: clinical recommendations*. St. Petersburg: Medpress.
6. **Nikolaeva, O. V.** (2016). *Psychological support of patients in dentistry: theory and practice*. Moscow: Stomatological School.
7. **Guriev, A. V.** (2021). *Long-term results of treatment of secondary deformities of the dentoalveolar system*. SPb.: Peter.
8. **Marchenko, V. L.** (2015). *Fundamentals of prosthetics in dentistry*. Moscow: Medicine.
9. **Frolova, T. I.** (2022). *Innovative technologies in diagnostics and treatment of stomatological diseases*. Moscow: Scientific World.
10. **Shevchuk, L. M.** (2020). *Retainers and their use after orthodontic treatment*. SPb.: Standard.

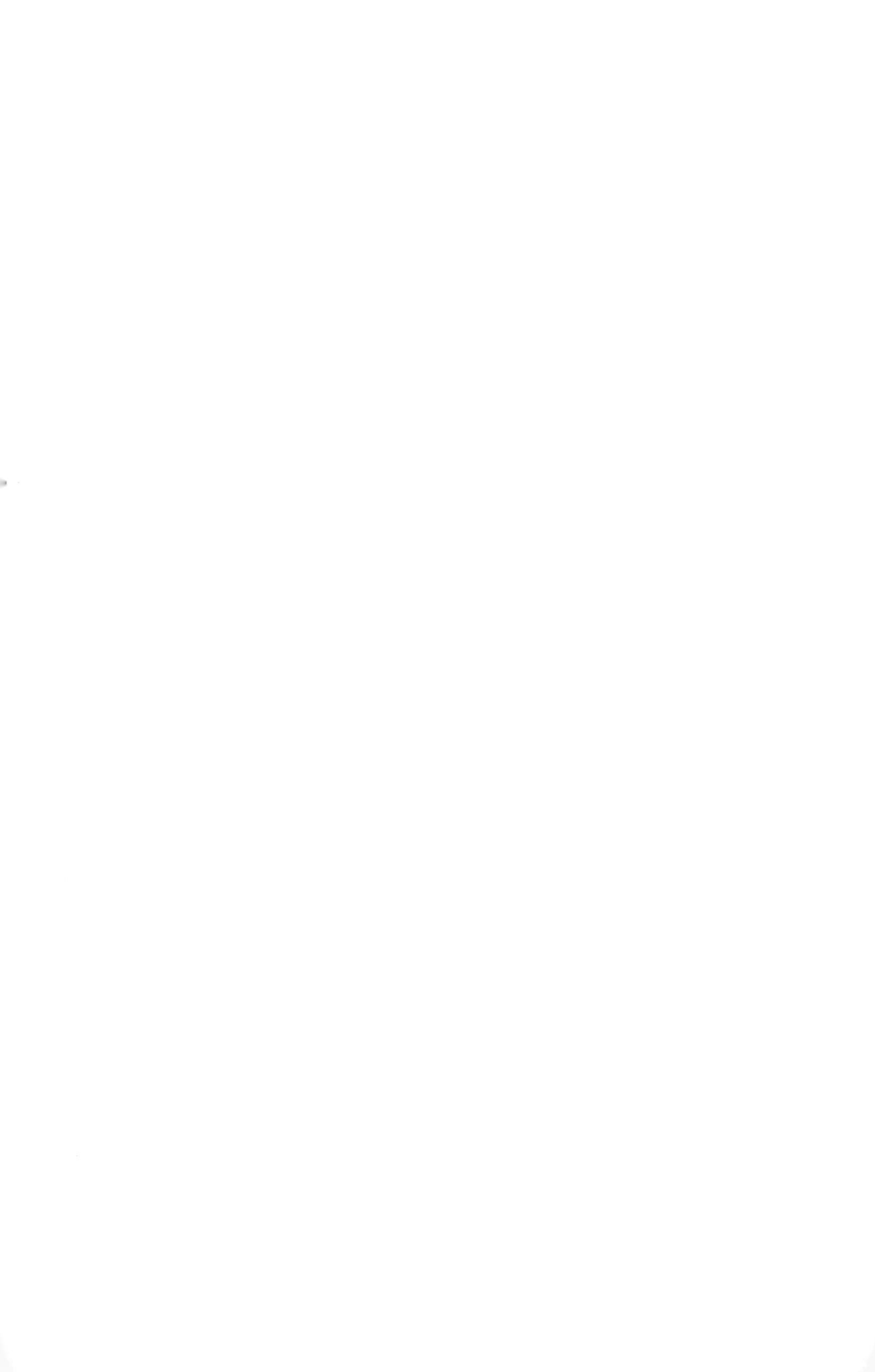

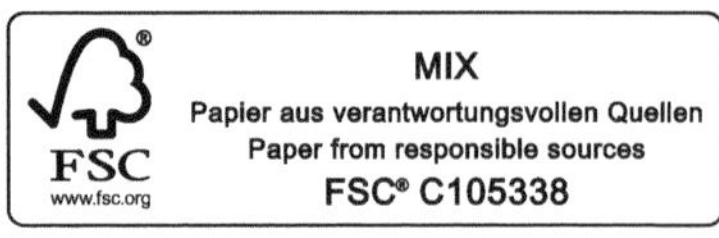

Printed by Books on Demand GmbH, Norderstedt / Germany